Aromatherapy

The complete guide to using aromatherapy and essential oils!

Table Of Contents

Introduction

I want to thank you and congratulate you for downloading the book, "Aromatherapy".

This book contains helpful information about aromatherapy, and how you can begin practicing it!

You will soon discover the different application methods of essential oils, and the benefits of each.

Provided in this book is a list of different oils, their benefits, and how to use them! You will also learn which essential oils mix well with each other, and what benefits this provides!

In no time you will be experiencing the full benefits of aromatherapy, and will be able to live a more relaxed and healthy life.

This book will explain to you tips and techniques that will allow you to successfully use aromatherapy to improve your health naturally from home!

I hope this book is able to help you, and wish you the best of luck with your aromatherapy experience!

Thanks again for downloading this book, I hope you enjoy it!

Chapter 1:
The Basics of Aromatherapy

What is Aromatherapy?

Aromatherapy is generally defined as the use of volatile plant oils, including essential oils, to enhance a person's physical and psychological wellbeing. It is considered to be an alternative or holistic form of medicine.

What are Essential Oils?

Essential oils are also sometimes called aromatherapy oils. They are basically the natural fragrant essences of plants, derived from the leaves, stems, bark, roots, flowers, and other parts.

How does Aromatherapy Work?

The use of aromatherapy oils promotes relaxation and stress relief. This allows the body to rejuvenate itself and heal itself better. The inhaled aromas are received by the olfactory receptors in the nasal cavity. Impulses are sent to the brain which stimulate the amygdale and the hippocampus. These are the parts of the brain that are responsible for our emotions and memories. Physical, emotional, mental, and psychological health can be influenced depending on the specific essential oil that is used.

What are the Benefits of Aromatherapy and Essential Oils?

1. Inhaling aromatherapy oils does not only trigger reactions in the brain. The inhaled natural components of the oils can have a therapeutic benefit when

breathing is concerned. For example, diffused eucalyptus oil can help to relieve airway congestion.

2. Diluted essential oils that are applied to the skin, can work to improve health, beauty, and hygiene. They can be used to alleviate the signs and symptoms of digestive problems, headaches, insomnia, and skin problems.

3. The use of aromatherapy oils can help to soothe and calm the body. This allows for the release of stress and tension.

4. Other uses for essential oils include being an ingredient for household cleaners, insect repellants, and insecticides.

Chapter 2:
Application Techniques and Methods for Essential Oils

There are many ways of using and applying essential oils. The methods that are used depend on a person's preference. Any of the methods can be used and a combination of them is effective as well.

Inhaling Essential Oils

1. Diffuser, Burner, Vaporizer: These devices use either water or heat to make essential oils evaporate.

2. Dry Evaporation: Several drops of an essential oil are placed on absorbent materials such as cotton balls or swabs and tissue papers. It is then allowed to naturally evaporate.

3. Steam Bath: One to two drops of an essential oil are mixed in a bowl or container of steaming water. Position your head above the steaming water and breathe in deeply. For a more potent effect, a towel can be placed over the head to keep the steam in.

4. Sprays: Several drops of an essential oil are mixed in with a water-based solution in a spray bottle. The mixtures can be sprayed to deodorize or to set a certain mood.

Other Essential Oil Application Techniques

1. Aromatherapy Baths: Several drops of an essential oil are mixed in to the bathwater.

2. Aromatherapy Massage Oils: Several drops of an essential oil are mixed in with a carrier lotion like shea butter, almond lotion, or cocoa butter.

3. Aromatherapy Massage: Several drops of an essential oil are mixed in with a carrier lotion like shea butter, almond lotion, or cocoa butter. A diluted essential oil mix can be used directly on the skin for the massage as well.

4. Aromatherapy Compress: Several drops of an essential oil are mixed in with warm water. A washcloth is dipped into the mixture and applied to the body. This method is especially useful for pain relief: menstrual cramps, headache, stomach ache, and muscle soreness.

Side note 1: There are other ways of using essential oils that are not necessarily beneficial due to their aromatherapy properties. One such way is through gargling. Several drops of an essential oil are mixed in with water. The solution is then used as a gargle.

Side note 2: There are some recipes that specify ingestion of essential oils but this should only be done with the advice and under the supervision of a trained aromatherapy practitioner. There are professionally prepared edible solutions of essential oils.

Chapter 3:
Preparation, Dilution, and Blending Essential Oils

Depending on the method chosen, the amount of essential oil used varies. Also for diluting, there is a specific ratio of the essential oil to its carrier oil.

Inhaled Essential Oils:

The essential oils are usually placed in devices such as burners, vaporizers, and diffusers. In general, the amount used for these devices is six drops of oil for one session. This amount can vary depending on the following factors:

- Type of device used

- Size of the room

- Age of the user

- Type of essential oil.

Essential Oils in Baths:

The usual amount of essential oils used in a bath is seven drops. It is best to do a skin test first if you have sensitive skin. The oils are added after you run the bath, and are mixed by hand.

For the elderly, and children aged four to twelve years, four drops of essential oils per bath is enough. Two drops of oil per bath is appropriate for pregnant women and children aged one to four years.

Essential Oils for Massage:

Note 1: Carrier oils are vegetable oils derived from the fat-rich portions of a plant, and are used to dilute essential oils.

Note 2: To use essential oils "neat" means to use them undiluted.

The amounts of essential oils listed below are mixed with twenty milliliters of carrier oil.

- Above sixty five years old: five drops

- Twelve to sixty five years old: ten drops

- Seven to eleven years old: seven drops

- Four to six years old: five drops

- One to three years old: two drops

- Under one year: one drop

- Pregnant Women: one drop

Essential Oils in Creams and Lotions:

The amounts of essential oils listed below are mixed with fifty grams of base cream or lotion.

- Above sixty five years old: ten drops

- Twelve to sixty five years old: twenty drops

- Four to eleven years old: ten drops

- One to three years old: four drops

- Under one year: two drops

- Pregnant Women: four drops

Essential Oils in Shampoos

The amounts of essential oils listed below are mixed with one hundred grams of shampoo.

- Above sixty five years old: ten drops

- Twelve to sixty five years old: twenty drops

- Four to eleven years old: ten drops

- One to three years old: two drops

- Under one year: not recommended

- Pregnant Women: five drops

Blending Essential Oils:

The blending and mixture of essential oils is based on their categories and notes. Some categories naturally blend well with others

Oils are categorized according to their aroma. Essential oils from the same categories usually blend together, but they can blend with oils from other categories as well.

The essential oil categories are:

- Floral: rose, lavender, and jasmine

- Earthy: patchouli and vetiver

- Woodsy: pine, spruce, and cedar

- Minty: peppermint and spearmint

- Herbaceous: marjoram, basil, and rosemary

- Spicy: clove, nutmeg, and cinnamon

- Citrus: orange, lemon, and lime

- Medicinal: tea tree oil and eucalyptus

- Oriental: ginger

The compatible categories for blending are:

- Floral with: citrus, spicy, and woodsy

- Woodsy with: all categories

- Spicy and oriental with: floral and citrus

- Minty with: earthy, herbaceous, woodsy, and citrus

Chapter 4:
Tips and Tricks for Aromatherapy Beginners

Aromatherapy may be complicated and confusing when first starting out. As with everything, practice makes perfect. Experimenting with different aromas and blending them according to your preference will become instinctive as time goes by. These tips are meant to help ease the process for aromatherapy beginners.

Choosing and Buying Essential Oils:

1. Perfume oils and essential oils are not the same. Perfumed oils do not have the same benefits as essential oils.

2. Be selective of where you buy your oils, and read up on the companies that sell them. The quality varies with each company and some products may not be as pure as the others.

3. Compare the ingredient labels of products with the same type of oil. For example, while two products may be labeled as lavender oil, the species of the plant they are gathered from may not be the same. The Latin name or botanical name is used to differentiate between similar products.

4. The quality and prices of the oils depends on the country of origin and species of the plant the oil was extracted from.

5. Take note of labels like: organic, ethically-farmed, and wild-crafted.

6. Be careful when purchasing products from street vendors, fair stalls, and craft shows.

7. On-line stores may sell high quality products at lower prices than local health food establishments.

Storage of Essential Oils:

1. Do not use bottles with rubber tops, stoppers, or droppers for storing essential oils. The concentrated oil can melt the rubber and turn it gummy. This can contaminate and ruin the oil.

2. Store your oils in dark tinted glass bottles preferably colored amber or cobalt blue. Keep them in a cool dark place away from direct sunlight.

Usage and Application of Essential Oils:

1. Only the smallest amount of oil that will get the job done effectively.

2. Some oils may not be safe to use during pregnancy. It is recommended to avoid them during the first trimester. Light use, about one percent dilution, is possible throughout the rest of the term. Safe oils for pregnancy include:

- Grapefruit

- Mandarin

- Tangerine

- Jasmine

- Geranium

- Ylang Ylang

3. The practice of aromatherapy is not limited to the use of pure essential oils.

Common Aromatherapy Products:

- Soaps, bath salts, shampoo

- Aromatherapy sprays and hydrosol mists

- Aromatic candles

- Incense sticks and cones

- Powder, lotions and creams

- Burning oils

- Blended massage oils

- Facial masks and body scrubs

- Balms and salves

Safety Guidelines and Precautions:

1. Always read the ingredient labels of aromatherapy products. Make sure to take note of warning labels and cautions.

2. As much as possible, avoid applying essential oils near the eye areas. If the oil comes in contact with the eye, flush it with large amounts of clean water. Running water from a tap can be used as well. Seek medical help when needed.

3. Keep essential oils and other aromatherapy products away from the reach of children. This is to prevent accidental ingestion that might lead to serious health-related complications.

4. Only use the suggested amount of oils needed and follow preparation instructions carefully. Misuse of aromatherapy techniques can cause headaches and some symptoms of nausea. When this happens, step out for some air and drink plenty of water.

5. Essential oils should be diluted before being directly applied to the skin. Undiluted concentrated oils can cause irritation and inflammation on the skin such as: itching, redness, swelling, and a burning sensation. If the undiluted oil accidentally comes in contact with the skin, wash the affected area under running water. Another option is to wash in warm and soapy water. Seek medical help when needed.

6. Unless specified for certain recipes, do not attempt to ingest essential oils. Seek medical help when this happens. It is also possible to drink and rinse out the mouth with milk to minimize the effect of the ingested oil.

7. Warning labels are put on for a reason. There are some oils that can cause allergies and can interfere with some medications. Some oils can be incompatible with certain health-related conditions, including epilepsy and hypotension.

8. Keep all essential oils away from potential fire hazards.

9. Keep the essential oils away from your eyes, nose, and
    ears.

10. When blending oils and making aromatherapy
    products, work in a well-ventilated room or area.

Chapter 5:
Aromatherapy Oil List

All aromatherapy oils have their own properties and specific use or benefit. They can be used as single oils or in blended mixtures. Below are lists of some of the most popular and commonly used aromatherapy oils.

Essential Oils:

Allspice Berry Oil

>   **Application Method:** aromatherapy massage, inhalation

>   **Uses and Benefits:** It evokes feelings of warmth, cheer, and comfort

>   **Blends Well With:** Ginger, Orange, Patchouli, Clove

>   **Precautions:** Some people may experience allergic reactions.

Amyris Oil

>   **Application Method:** aromatherapy massage, inhalation

>   **Uses and Benefits:** It evokes feelings of strength and being centered

>   **Blends Well With:** cedar wood, rose, jasmine

>   **Precautions:** Some people may experience allergic reactions.

Anise Oil

>   **Application Method:** aromatherapy massage, inhalation

Uses and Benefits: It evokes feelings of cheer and euphoria

Precautions: Some people may experience allergic reactions.

Basil Oil

Application Method: aromatherapy massage, inhalation

Uses and Benefits: It is clarifying, refreshing, and energizing

Blends Well With: clary sage, lime oil, bergamot

Precautions: Some people may experience allergic reactions.

Bay Oil

Application Method: aromatherapy massage, inhalation

Uses and Benefits: Evokes feelings of warmth and clarity

Precautions: Some people may experience allergic reactions.

Bergamot Oil

Application Methods: incense, vaporizers, baths, as massage oil

Uses and Benefits:

1. Treatment for:

- Stress

- Anxiety

- Depression

- Anorexia

- Psoriasis

- Eczema

2. Stimulation for: liver, spleen, and digestive system

3. Pick-me-up for people with generalized body malaise

Precautions:

- Applying the pure form of the oil directly to the skin can cause burns, especially when exposed to sunlight.

- It is advisable to use stay away from direct sunlight when using bergamot oil.

Birch Oil

Application Method: aromatherapy massage

Uses and Benefits: Relief for muscle pain and body stiffness

Precautions: Some people may experience allergic reactions.

Camphor Oil (white)

Application Method: aromatherapy massage, inhalation

Uses and Benefits: It is clarifying, energizing, and purifying

Precautions: Some people may experience allergic reactions.

Cardamom Seed Oil

Application Method: aromatherapy massage, inhalation

Uses and Benefits: It evokes feelings of warmth, comfort, and allure

Blends Well With: ylang ylang, cedarwood, frankincense, bergamot

Precautions: Some people may experience allergic reactions.

Carrot Seed Oil

Application Method: aromatherapy massage, inhalation

Uses and Benefits:

1. It evokes feelings of nourishment and rejuvenation

2. For skin care

Precautions: Some people may experience allergic reactions.

Cassia Bark Oil

Application Method: aromatherapy massage, inhalation

Uses and Benefits:

1. It evokes feelings of warmth and comfort

2. As an energizing agent

Precautions: It can be irritating when undiluted.

Cedar Oil

Application Method: aromatherapy massage, inhalation

Uses and Benefits: It evokes feelings of strength, stability, and being centered.

Precautions: Some people may experience allergic reactions.

Cedar wood Oil

Application Method: as a massage oil, vapor inhalation, mixed with facial creams

Uses and Benefits:

1. Relieves stress and anxiety

2. Helps with respiratory problems and skin-related problems

Precautions: It is not recommended for pregnant women. Undiluted cedar wood oil can cause skin irritation.

Chamomile Oil

Application Method: as a massage oil, steam or vapor inhalation, mixed with creams and lotions

Uses and Benefits:

1. As a calming agent

2. For improvement of mood and antidepressant

Precautions: It is not recommended for pregnant women and for people with allergies to ragweed.

Cinnamon Oil

Application Method: as a massage oil, mixed with creams and lotions

Uses and Benefits: For reducing drowsiness and irritability

Precautions: Some people may experience allergic reactions.

Citronella Oil

Application Method: aromatherapy massage, inhalation

Uses and Benefits: It is revitalizing and purifying

Precautions: Some people may experience allergic reactions.

Clary Sage Oil

Application Method: as a massage oil, mixed with creams and lotions

Uses and Benefits: For relief of muscle tension

Precautions: Some people may experience allergic reactions.

Clove Oil

Application Method: as a massage oil, mixed with creams and lotions

Uses and Benefits:

1. As an antiseptic

2. For pain relief

Precautions: Some people may experience allergic reactions.

Coriander Seed Oil

Application Method: aromatherapy massage, inhalation

Uses and Benefits: It evokes feelings of being nurtured and being supported

Blends Well With: cinnamon bark, frankincense, bergamot, jasmine, clary sage

Cypress Oil

Application Method: aromatherapy massage

Uses and Benefits: Treatment for hypotension and poor blood circulation

Precautions: Some people may experience allergic reactions.

Eucalyptus Oil

Application Method: inhalation, as massage oil

Uses and Benefits:

1. To enhance concentration

2. As decongestant and relief for various respiratory problems

3. As an antiseptic

4. As a deodorizing agent

5. Treatment for migraine, fever, body aches, and muscle pains

Precautions: It is not recommended for pregnant and lactating women as well as for people suffering from epilepsy. Ingestion of large amounts can be fatal.

Fennel Oil

Application Method: aromatherapy massage, inhalation

Uses and Benefits: It evokes feelings of rejuvenation, nurturing, and being supported.

Precautions: Some people may experience allergic reactions.

Fir Oil

Application Method: inhalation and aromatherapy massage

Uses and Benefits:

1. As a deodorizing agent

2. As a soothing and calming agent

3. To relieve muscle pains and rheumatism

Precautions: Some people may experience allergic reactions.

Frankincense Oil

Application Method: aromatherapy massage, inhalation

Uses and Benefits:

1. It is a calming agent

2. It gives way to a meditative state

Precautions: Some people may experience allergic reactions.

Geranium Oil

Application Method: aromatherapy massage

Uses and Benefits: For treatment of skin related problems

Precautions: Some people may experience allergic reactions.

Ginger Oil

Application Method: inhalation and aromatherapy massage

Uses and Benefits:

1. Appetite stimulant

2. To relieve headaches

Precautions: Some people may experience allergic reactions.

Grapefruit Oil

Application Method: aromatherapy massage, inhalation, mixed with creams and lotions

Uses and Benefits: It is refreshing and cheering

Precautions: Some people may experience allergic reactions.

Hyssop Oil

Application Method: aromatherapy massage, inhalation

Uses and Benefits: It is refreshing and purifying

Blends Well With: clary sage, myrtle, lavender, clove, rosemary, and citrus oils

Precautions: Some people may experience allergic reactions.

Jasmine Oil

Application Method: inhalation, as massage oil, aromatherapy bath

Uses and Benefits:

1. To help ease depression

2. To enhance libido

3. To reduce stress and tension

4. To help relieve respiratory problems

Precautions: It is not recommended for pregnant women.

Juniper Berry Oil

Application Method: aromatherapy massage

Uses and Benefits: Treatment for arthritis and varicose veins

Precautions: Some people may experience allergic reactions.

Lavender Oil

Application Method: inhalation, as massage oil, aromatherapy bath

Uses and Benefits:

1. For stress relief

2. As a relaxing agent

3. To help relieve sleeping troubles

4. As an antidepressant and sedative

5. As a deodorizing agent

Precautions: Some people may experience allergic reactions.

Lemon Oil

Application Method: inhalation, mixed in lotions or creams, aromatherapy bath

Uses and Benefits:

1. For improvement of concentration

2. Helps with better digestion

3. Relieves arthritic pain

4. Helps boost the immune system

5. Helps to relieve skin irritation

6. As a mood enhancer

7. To treat headaches and fevers

Precautions: Some people may experience allergic reactions. It is advisable to keep away from direct sunlight as well.

Lemongrass Oil

Application Method: inhalation, mixed in lotions or creams, aromatherapy bath

Uses and Benefits:

1. As a deodorizing agent

2. For pain relief

Precautions: Some people may experience allergic reactions.

Lime Oil

Application Method: aromatherapy massage, inhalation

Uses and Benefits:

1. It is refreshing and cheering.

2. Used as a deodorizing agent

Precautions: Exposure to sunlight after usage can cause skin irritation.

Marjoram Oil

Application Method: inhalation, aromatherapy bath, massage

Uses and Benefits:

1. To calm hyperactivity

2. For relief of fatigue, anxiety and stress

3. Helps to alleviate depression

4. Treatment for cramps, tension, and, headaches

5. Treatment for sinusitis and asthma

6. For relief of insomnia

Precautions: It is not recommended for pregnant women.

Myrtle Oil

Application Method: aromatherapy massage, inhalation

Uses and Benefits: It is clarifying and cleansing.

Blends Well With: clary sage, lime oil, bergamot, rosemary, lavender

Precautions: Some people may experience allergic reactions.

Myrrh Oil

Application Method: inhalation, massage oil

Uses and Benefits: Treatment for dry, chapped, and aging skin

Precautions: Some people may experience allergic reactions.

Neroli Oil

Application Method: as a massage oil, mixed with creams and lotions

Uses and Benefits: For improvement of blood circulation and skin health

Precautions: Some people may experience allergic reactions.

Nutmeg Oil

Application Method: aromatherapy massage, inhalation

Uses and Benefits: It is energizing, uplifting, and rejuvenating

Precautions: Some people may experience allergic reactions.

Orange Oil

Application Method: as a massage oil, mixed with creams and lotions

Uses and Benefits:

1. To alter moods

2. As a deodorizing agent

3. Helps to lower blood pressure

Precautions: Some people may experience allergic reactions.

Oregano Oil

Application Method: aromatherapy massage, inhalation

Uses and Benefits: It is invigorating, uplifting, and purifying.

Precautions: Some people may experience allergic reactions.

Palmarosa Oil

Application Method: aromatherapy massage, aromatherapy bath, mixed with creams and lotions

Uses and Benefits:

1. It is refreshing

2. It is used as a cleanser and astringent

Precautions: Some people may experience allergic reactions.

Patchouli Oil

Application Method: inhalation, aromatherapy bath, aromatherapy massage, mixed with lotions and creams

Uses and Benefits:

1. As a mood lifter

2. Alleviates fatigue, depression, and anxiety

3. For treatment of skin infections and wounds

4. As a skin care agent

Precautions: Some people may experience allergic reactions.

Peppermint Oil

Application Method: inhalation, aromatherapy bath, aromatherapy massage, mixed with lotions and creams

Uses and Benefits:

To enhance mental alertness

1. As an energy booster

2. As a mood enhancer

3. To relieve congestion

Precautions: It is not for recommended for pregnant women. Keep away from the eye areas.

Pine Oil

Application Method: aromatherapy massage, aromatherapy bath, mixed with creams and lotions

Uses and Benefits:

- It is used as a deodorizing agent

- It is refreshing and invigorating

Precautions: Some people may experience allergic reactions, especially when it is undiluted.

Rose Oil

Application Method: inhalation, aromatherapy bath, aromatherapy massage, mixed with lotions and creams

Uses and Benefits:

1. Helps with depression

2. Relieves anxiety

Precautions: It is not for recommended for pregnant women.

Rosemary Oil

Application Method: inhalation, aromatherapy bath, aromatherapy massage, mixed with lotions and creams, mixed with shampoos

Uses and Benefits:

1. As a mental stimulant and memory booster

2. Relieves sinusitis and congestion

3. Relieves muscle pain, arthritic pain, and digestive disorders

4. For stimulation of the scalp and hair growth

Precautions: It is not for recommended for pregnant women and people with epilepsy and hypertension.

Rosewood Oil

Application Method: inhalation, aromatherapy bath, aromatherapy massage, mixed with lotions and creams

Uses and Benefits: It is relaxing, sensual, and centering.

Precautions: Watch out for any allergic reactions.

Sandalwood Oil

Application Method: inhalation, incense, mixed with lotions and creams

Uses and Benefits:

1. Relieves chest pain

2. Relieves stress and promotes relaxation

3. For skin hydration

Precautions: Some people may experience allergic reactions.

Spearmint Oil

Application Method: inhalation, aromatherapy bath

Uses and Benefits: It is refreshing, cooling, and revitalizing.

Precautions: Watch out for any allergic reactions.

Spruce Oil

Application Method: inhalation, aromatherapy bath, mixed with creams and lotions

Uses and Benefits:

1. It is clarifying and revitalizing.

2. Used as a disinfectant

3. Used as a deodorizing agent

Blends well with: cedar wood, rosemary, pine oils, and galbanum

Precautions: Watch out for any allergic reactions.

Tangerine Oil

Application Method: inhalation, aromatherapy bath

Uses and Benefits:

1. It is cheering and uplifting.

2. Used as a deodorizing agent

Precautions: Watch out for any allergic reactions.

Tea Tree Oil

Application Method: inhalation, massage, mixed with lotions and creams, aromatherapy bath, mixed in shampoos

Uses and Benefits:

1. Boosts the immune system

2. For skin healing

3. As an insecticide

4. Treatment of:

   - Cold sores

   - Muscle pain

   - Respiratory conditions including flu

   - Athlete's foot

   - Dandruff

Blends well with: rosemary and nutmeg oils

Precautions: Avoid contact with the eyes and do not use near deep cuts.

Thyme Oil

Application Method: massage, mixed with lotions and creams

Uses and Benefits: To fight infections

Precautions: Some people may have allergic reactions.

Vanilla Oil

Application Method: inhalation, aromatherapy bath

Uses and Benefits: It is calming, comforting, and balancing

Precautions: Watch out for any allergic reactions.

Vetiver Oil

Application Method: inhalation, aromatherapy bath

Uses and Benefits:

1. It is supportive and grounding

2. Used as a perfume and deodorizer

Precautions: Watch out for any allergic reactions.

Wintergreen Oil

Application Method: inhalation, aromatherapy bath

Uses and Benefits: It is refreshing and invigorating

Precautions: Watch out for any allergic reactions.

Ylang Ylang Oil

Application Method: inhalation, massage, mixed with lotions and creams, aromatherapy bath, mixed with shampoos

Uses and Benefits:

1. For stress relief

2. As an aphrodisiac

3. As a calming agent

4. A scalp stimulant for hair growth

5. Treatment for:

    - Headaches

    - Nausea

    - Skin conditions

    - Hypertension

    - Intestinal problems

Precautions: Overuse of the oil can cause headaches.

List of Common Carrier Oils:

1. Coconut Oil

2. Olive Oil

3. Jojoba Oil

4. Safflower Oil

5. Sweet Almond Oil

6. Apricot Kernel Oil

7. Peanut Oil

8. Macadamia Nut Oil

9. Cranberry Seed Oil

10. Avocado Oil

11. Grape Seed Oil

12. Hemp Seed Oil

13. Hazelnut Oil

14. Borage Seed Oil

15. Camelia Seed Oil

16. Evening Primrose Oil

17. Pecan Oil

18. Rose Hip Oil

19. Pomegranate Oil

20.Sesame Oil

21. Sunflower Oil

22.Watermelon Seed Oil

List of Essential Oils to Avoid:

1. Bitter Almond Oil

2. Mugwort Oil

3. Horseradish Oil

4. Calamus Oil

5. Mustard Oil

6. Savin Oil

7. Yellow Camphor Oil

8. Rue Oil

9. Tansy Oil

10. Southernwood Oil

Chapter 6:
Practical Home Uses of Aromatherapy

Aromatherapy is not only limited to the application of oils on the body, or using devices to diffuse them for inhalation. Essential oils can be used for other things in practical ways around the house. The following list contains suggestions for practical aromatherapy at home.

1. **Daytime Shower:** Three to six drops of any citrus oil placed on the shower floor can be very refreshing.

2. **Nighttime Shower**: Lavender oils and chamomile oils can help you to relax before bedtime.

3. **Making use of the radiator**: One good way to give a nice aroma to any room is to put a few drops of oil on a piece of tissue paper that is put over the radiator.

4. **Car Fresheners**: A few drops of essential oils such as peppermint can be sprinkled on the car's carpet floor to keep it smelling fresh.

5. **Keeping mattresses fresh**: About ten to twenty drops of essential oils sprinkled on a mattress will help to freshen it and keep it clean. Recommended oils are lavender and tea tree.

6. **Keeping clothes fresh**: Misting clothes with lavender water on the clothes while ironing will keep them smelling fresh.

7. **For dish cloths:** Adding several drops of lemon oil on a dish rag will help to keep it disinfected, and free from harmful microorganisms.

8. **Refrigerator:** Wiping the outer surfaces of the fridge with a cloth dipped in lemon oil water will help to remove unwanted odors.

9. **Mops**: Four to six drops of citrusy essential oils added to the mop bucket will keep it smelling clean and fresh.

10. **Bathrooms, closets, and attics**: Placing a cotton ball dipped in essential oils in a glass bowl, and positioning it in the room can help to dispel unpleasant smells.

11. **Air fresheners**: An empty spray bottle or an atomizer can be filled with a mixture of water and essential oils. About five milliliters of oil in one hundred milliliters of water is enough to make a good spray.

    - **Common rooms:** lemon, orange, grapefruit, or bergamot

    - **Bedrooms:** chamomile or lavender

    - **Sickrooms:** lemon oils and tea tress

    - **Study room or library:** rosemary or basil

    - **Party rooms:** orange, sandalwood, or ylang ylang oils

12. **Other places to sprinkle essential oils:**

    - Inside of old shoes

    - Clean carpets, mats, and rugs

    - Table centerpieces during special occasions

- Couch pillows

- Bathroom and washroom hand towels

Conclusion

Thank you again for downloading this book!

I hope this book was able to help you learn more about aromatherapy!

Try out as many of the different oils as you can, and experiment with different mixtures and techniques to see what you like best!

The next step is to put this information to use, and begin using aromatherapy in your life!

Finally, if you enjoyed this book, please take the time to share your thoughts and post a review on Amazon. It'd be greatly appreciated!

Thank you and good luck!

www.ingramcontent.com/pod-product-compliance
Lightning Source LLC
Chambersburg PA
CBHW051737050726
47598CB00003B/1227